HEART FAILURE

Unique Guide on Heart Failures, Its Types, Causes, Complications and Prevention

Dr. Charles Rex

Table of Contents

CHAPTER ONE 3
  BASICS OF HEART FAILURE 3
  SYMPTOMS 5

CHAPTER TWO 8
  SIGNS TO SEE A DOCTOR 8
  CAUSES 10

CHAPTER THREE 14
  TYPE OF CORONARY FAILURE 14
    LEFT-SIDED CORONARY FAILURE 14
    RIGHT-SIDED CORONARY FAILURE 14
    SYSTOLIC CORONARY CORONARY FAILURE 14

CHAPTER FOUR 21
  CAUSES OF ACUTE CORONARY FAILURE 21
  COMPLICATIONS 27
  PREVENTION 30
  THE END 32

CHAPTER ONE

BASICS OF HEART FAILURE

Heart failure, sometimes referred to as congestive coronary coronary failure, occurs while your cardiac muscle doesn't pump blood also because it need to. Certain conditions, along side narrowed arteries in your coronary heart (coronary artery ailment) or high blood strain, progressively get away your heart too weak or stiff to fill and pump successfully.

Not all conditions that cause coronary coronary

failure are often reversed, but remedies can improve the signs and symptoms and signs and symptoms of coronary failure and assist you reside longer. Lifestyle adjustments — which include exercising, lowering sodium on your diet, handling strain and dropping weight — can improve your excellent of life. One manner to stop coronary coronary
failure is to save lots of you and manage situations that purpose coronary
failure, alongside arteria
coronaria sickness, high vital

sign, diabetes or obesity.

SYMPTOMS

Heart failureOpen pop-up conversation box Heart failure are often ongoing (chronic), or your condition can also start suddenly (acute). Heart failure signs and symptoms and signs can also encompass:

- Shortness of breath (dyspnea) once you exert your self or while you lie
- Fatigue and weakness
- Swelling (edema) on your legs,

ankles and feet
- Rapid or irregular heartbeat
- Reduced ability to exercise
- Persistent cough or wheezing with white or pink blood-tinged phlegm
- Increased want to urinate in the dark
- Swelling of your abdomen (ascites)
- in no time weight gain from fluid retention
- Lack of urge for food and nausea
- Difficulty concentrating or reduced alertness
- Sudden, excessive shortness of breath and expulsion purple,

foamy mucus
- Chest ache just in case your coronary coronary failure is resulting from a coronary attack

CHAPTER TWO

SIGNS TO SEE A DOCTOR

See your doctor if you think that you is perhaps experiencing signs and symptoms or symptoms of coronary failure. Seek emergency remedy if you enjoy any of the following:
- Chest ache
- Fainting or extreme weakness
- Rapid or abnormal heartbeat associated
with shortness of breath, pain or fainting
- Sudden, extreme shortness of breath and expulsion pink, foamy

mucus

Although these signs and symptoms and symptoms are often thanks to coronary failure , there are numerous other feasible reasons, which include other life-threatening coronary heart and lung situations. Don't attempt to diagnose yourself. Call your local emergency number for immediate help. ER docs will attempt to stabilize your circumstance and choose if your signs and symptoms are thanks to coronary coronary failure or something else. If you've got a prognosis of coronary coronary failure and if any of the symptoms suddenly grow to be worse otherwise you develop a replacement signal or symptom, it's ready to imply that present coronary failure is getting worse or not responding to remedy. this will be also the case just in case you benefit 5 pounds (2.3 kg) or more within a couple of days. Contact your doctor promptly.

CAUSES

Heart failure regularly develops after other situations have damaged or weakened your heart. However, the guts don't want to be weakened to reason coronary failure. It can additionally arise if the coronary heart will become too stiff. In coronary failure, the first pumping chambers of your coronary heart (the ventricles) may find yourself stiff and not fill well between beats. During a few instances of coronary failure, your cardiac muscle may additionally grow to be broken and weakened, and therefore the ventricles stretch (dilate) to the purpose that the guts can't pump blood successfully throughout your body. Over time, the coronary heart can't continue with the everyday demands positioned thereon to pump blood to the relief of your body. An ejection fraction is a critical measurement of how properly your coronary heart is pumping and is employed to help classify coronary failure and guide remedy. During a healthy heart, the ejection fraction is 50 percent or higher — which suggests that quite half of the blood that fills the ventricle is pumped out with every beat. But coronary failure can arise despite an ordinary ejection fraction. This happens if the guts muscle turns into stiff from situations consisting of excessive vital sign. Heart failure can contain the left side (left ventricle), right side (right ventricle) or each side of your heart. Generally, coronary failure begins with the left side, particularly the ventricle — your heart's most vital pumping chamber.

CHAPTER THREE

TYPE OF CORONARY FAILURE

LEFT-SIDED CORONARY FAILURE
Fluid may additionally returned abreast of your lungs, inflicting shortness of breath.

RIGHT-SIDED CORONARY FAILURE
Fluid may additionally lower copy into your abdomen, legs and feet, causing swelling.

SYSTOLIC CORONARY CORONARY FAILURE
The ventricle can't agreement vigorously, indicating a pumping problem.

DIASTOLIC CORONARY FAILURE (additionally referred to as coronary coronary failure with preserved ejection fraction) The ventricle can't relax or fill fully, indicating a filling problem. Any of the subsequent situations can harm or weaken your heart and may purpose coronary failure. A number of these could also be present without your knowing it:

• arteria coronaria sickness and coronary attack. Arteria coronaria ailment is that the commonest place shape of heart sickness and therefore the most common purpose of coronary failure. The ailment outcomes from the buildup of fatty deposits (plaque) on your arteries, which lessen blood float and may end in coronary attack.

• High blood strain (hypertension). If your vital sign is excessive, your heart has got to work tougher than it need to circulate blood at some stage in your body. Over time, this greater exertion could make your cardiac muscle too stiff or too vulnerable to efficiently pump blood.

• Faulty coronary heart valves. The valves of your heart maintain blood flowing within the right path thru the coronary heart. A broken valve — thanks to a coronary heart defect, arteria coronaria disease or coronary heart infection — forces your heart to figure harder, which could weaken it over time.

- Damage to the guts muscle (cardiomyopathy). Cardiac muscle damage (cardiomyopathy) could have many reasons, including numerous diseases, infections, alcoholic abuse and therefore the toxic impact of tablets, like cocaine or some capsules used for chemotherapy.

Genetic elements can also play a task.

• Myocarditis. Myocarditis is an infection of the guts muscle. It's most typically due to an epidemic, which incorporates COVID-19, and may cause left-sided coronary failure.

• Heart defects you're born with (congenital coronary heart defects). If your coronary heart and its chambers or valves haven't fashioned correctly, the healthful elements of your heart need to work tougher to pump blood thru your coronary heart, which, in turn, also can cause coronary failure.

• Abnormal heart rhythms (coronary heart arrhythmias). Abnormal heart rhythms may additionally motive your heart to beat too fast, creating more work to your heart. A sluggish heartbeat also may additionally end
in coronary failure

• Other diseases. Chronic diseases — alongside diabetes, HIV, hyperthyroidism, hypothyroidism, or a buildup of iron (hemochromatosis) or protein (amyloidosis) — additionally may additionally contribute to failure.

CHAPTER FOUR

CAUSES OF ACUTE CORONARY FAILURE

Coronary failure encompass viruses that attack the coronary cardiac muscle, intense infections, allergies, blood clots inside the lungs, using certain medicines or any illness that affects the entire body. A single chance factor is often sufficient to cause coronary failure, but a mixture of things also will increase your hazard.

Risk factors consist of:
- High vital sign. Your coronary

heart works tougher than it's to just in case your vital sign is excessive.

• arteria coronaria disease. Narrowed arteries may additionally restrict your coronary heart's deliver of oxygen-wealthy blood, ensuing in weakened cardiac muscle.

• Heart assault. A heart assault may be a shape of coronary ailment that happens suddenly. Damage on your coronary cardiac muscle from a coronary attack may additionally imply your coronary heart cannot pump also because it should.

- Diabetes. Having diabetes will increase your hazard of high blood stress and arteria coronaria disease.
- Some diabetes medicinal drugs. The diabetes capsules rosiglitazone (Avandia) and pioglitazone (Actos) are discovered to growth the prospect of coronary coronary failure during a few people. Don't forestall taking these medicinal drugs in your own, though. If you are taking them, speak together with your physician whether or not you would like to form any modifications.

- Certain medications. Some medicines can also cause coronary failure or coronary heart issues. Medications which may also boom the hazard of coronary heart problems encompass nonsteroidal anti-inflammatory drug drugs (NSAIDs); positive anesthesia medications; a couple of anti-arrhythmic medications; certain medicines wont to treat high blood strain, cancer, blood conditions, neurological situations, psychiatric situations, lung situations, urological situations, inflammatory situations and infections; and other prescription and over-the-counter medicines. Don't forestall taking any medications to your own. If you've got questions on medicines you are taking, ask your health practitioner whether he or she recommends any changes.

• Apnea. The lack to breathe properly while you sleep in the dark are causes of low blood oxygen degrees and increased hazard of atypical coronary heart rhythms. Both of those troubles can weaken the guts.

• Congenital heart defects.

Some those that expand coronary coronary failure were born with structural heart defects.

• Valvular heart sickness. People with valvular heart ailment have a better chance of coronary coronary failure.

• Viruses. A viral contamination also can have broken your cardiac muscle.

• Alcohol use. Drinking an excessive amount of alcohol can weaken coronary cardiac muscle and end
in coronary coronary failure.

• Tobacco use. Using tobacco can grow your risk of coronary

failure.

• Obesity. People that are obese have a better danger of growing coronary failure.

• Irregular heartbeats. These atypical rhythms, specifically if they're quite common and fast, can weaken the guts muscle and cause coronary coronary failure.

COMPLICATIONS

If you've coronary failure, your outlook relies upon on the rationale and therefore the severity, your ordinary health, and other factors alongside your age. Complications can encompass:

- Kidney harm or failure. Coronary failure can reduce the blood float on your kidneys, which may finally motive renal failure if left untreated. Kidney harm from coronary coronary failure can require dialysis for remedy.
- Heart valve issues. The valves of your coronary heart, which preserve blood flowing within the proper route through your heart, won't function well just in case your heart is enlarged or if the strain for your coronary heart is extremely high thanks

to coronary failure.

• Cardiac rhythm troubles. Cardiac rhythm problems (arrhythmias) could also be a capacity difficulty of coronary failure.

• Liver damage. Coronary failure can cause a buildup of fluid that puts an excessive amount of pressure at the liver. This fluid backup may result in scarring, which makes it extra difficult for your liver to characteristic properly. Some people's signs and symptoms and heart feature will improve with proper treatment.

However, coronary failure could also be life-threatening. People with coronary failure may have severe signs and symptoms, and a couple of can also require heart transplantation or help with a ventricular assist device.

PREVENTION

The key to stopping coronary failure is to reduce your danger elements. You'll control or do away with many the hazard elements for coronary heart ailment — high vital sign and arteria coronaria disorder, for instance — via making lifestyle changes at the side of the assist of any wished medicinal drugs. Lifestyle modifications you'll make to help prevent coronary failure include:

- Not smoking
- Controlling sure conditions, which include high blood strain and diabetes
- Staying physically active
- Eating healthy foods
- Maintaining a wholesome weight
- Reducing and dealing with strain

THE END

www.ingramcontent.com/pod-product-compliance
Lightning Source LLC
Chambersburg PA
CBHW050307220526
45465CB00002B/866